The Best Keto Chaffle Cooking Guide

50 Delicious Keto Chaffle Recipes for Tasty Meals

Kade Harrison

Table of Contents

Delicious Bagel Chaffle

Preparation time:

10 minutes

Cooking time:

8 minutes

Servings: 2

Ingredients:

- 1 egg, lightly beaten
- 1/4 tsp garlic powder
- 1/4 tsp onion powder
- 1 1/2 tsp bagel seasoning
- 3/4 cup mozzarella cheese, shredded
- 1/2 tsp baking powder, gluten-free
- 1 tbsp almond flour

Directions:

1. Preheat your waffle maker.
2. In a bowl, mix egg, bagel seasoning, baking powder, onion powder, garlic powder, and almond flour until well combined.
3. Add cheese and stir well.
4. Spray waffle maker with cooking spray.

5. Pour 1/2 of batter in the hot waffle maker and cook for 5 minutes or until golden brown.
6. Repeat with the remaining batter.
7. Serve and enjoy.

Cheesy Garlic Bread Chaffle

Preparation time:

10 minutes

Cooking time:

8 minutes

Servings: 2

Ingredients:

- 1 egg, lightly beaten
- 1 tsp parsley, minced
- 2 tbsp parmesan cheese, grated
- 1 tbsp butter, melted
- 1/4 tsp garlic powder
- 1/4 tsp baking powder, gluten-free
- 1 tsp coconut flour
- 1/2 cup cheddar cheese, shredded

Directions:

1. Preheat your waffle maker.
2. In a bowl, whisk egg, garlic powder, baking powder, coconut flour, and cheddar cheese until well combined.
3. Spray waffle maker with cooking spray.
4. Pour half of the batter in the hot waffle maker and cook for 3 minutes or until set. Repeat with the remaining batter.
5. Brush chaffles with melted butter.

6. Place chaffles on baking tray and top with parmesan cheese and broil until cheese melted.
7. Garnish with parsley and serve.

Zucchini Basil Chaffle

Preparation time:

10 minutes

Cooking time:

8 minutes

Servings: 2

Ingredients:

- 1 egg, lightly beaten
- 1/4 cup fresh basil, chopped
- 1/4 cup mozzarella cheese, shredded
- 1/2 cup parmesan cheese, shredded
- 1 cup zucchini, grated and squeeze out all liquid
- 1/4 tsp pepper
- 3/4 tsp salt

Directions:

1. Preheat your waffle maker.
2. In a small bowl, beat the egg.
3. Add basil, mozzarella cheese, zucchini, pepper, and salt and stir well.
4. Spray waffle maker with cooking spray.
5. Sprinkle 2 tbsp of parmesan cheese to the bottom of waffle iron then spread 1/4 of the batter and top with

2 tbsp parmesan cheese and cook for 4-8 minutes or until set. Repeat with the remaining batter.

6. Serve and enjoy.

Jicama Chaffle

Preparation time:

10 minutes

Cooking time:

8 minutes

Servings: 2

Ingredients:

- 2 eggs, lightly beaten
- 1 cup cheddar cheese, shredded
- 1/4 tsp garlic powder
- 1/4 tsp onion powder
- 1 large jicama root, peel, shredded and squeeze out all liquid
- Pepper
- Salt

Directions:

1. Preheat your waffle maker.
2. Add shredded jicama in microwave-safe bowl and microwave for 5-8 minutes.
3. Add remaining ingredients to the bowl and stir to combine.
4. Spray waffle maker with cooking spray.
5. Pour half of the batter in the hot waffle maker and cook until golden

brown or set. Repeat with the remaining batter.

6. Serve and enjoy.

Bacon & Chicken Ranch Chaffle

Preparation Time:

5 minutes

Cooking Time:

8 minutes

Servings: 2

Ingredients:

- 1 egg
- ¼ cup chicken cubes, cooked
- 1 slice bacon, cooked and chopped
- ¼ cup cheddar cheese, shredded
- 1 teaspoon ranch dressing powder

Directions:

1. Preheat your waffle maker.
2. In a bowl, mix all the ingredients.
3. Add half of the mixture to your waffle maker.
4. Cover and cook for 4 minutes.
5. Make the second chaffle using the same steps.

Pumpkin & Pecan Chaffle

Preparation Time:

5 minutes

Cooking Time:

10 minutes

Servings: 2

Ingredients:

- 1 egg, beaten
- ½ cup mozzarella cheese, grated
- ½ teaspoon pumpkin spice
- 1 tablespoon pureed pumpkin
- 2 tablespoons almond flour
- 1 teaspoon sweetener
- 2 tablespoons pecans, chopped

Directions:

1. Turn on the waffle maker.
2. Beat the egg in a bowl.
3. Stir in the rest of the ingredients.
4. Pour half of the mixture into the device.
5. Seal the lid.
6. Cook for 5 minutes.
7. Remove the chaffle carefully.

8. Repeat the steps to make the second chaffle.

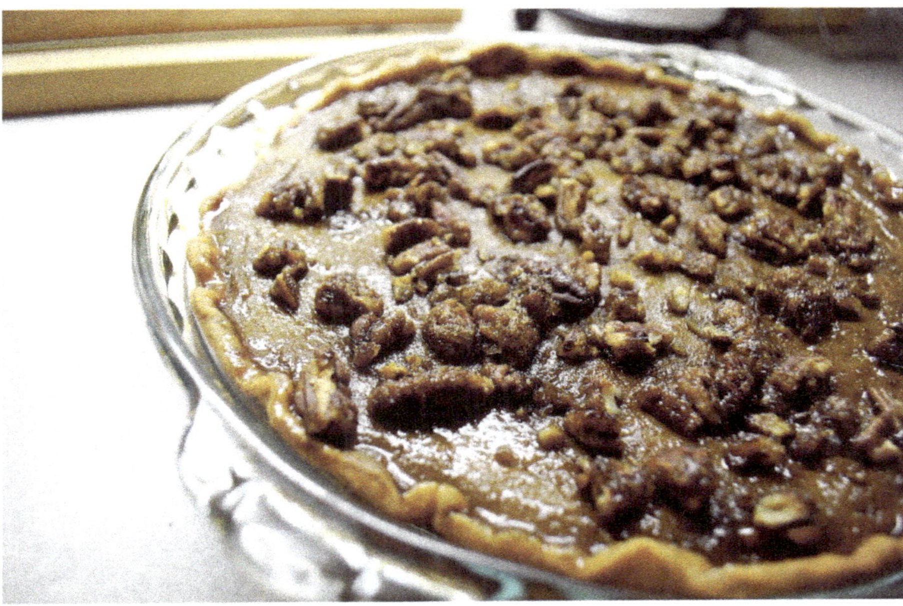

Cheeseburger Chaffle

Preparation Time:

15 minutes

Cooking Time:

15 minutes

Servings: 2

Ingredients:

- 1 lb. ground beef
- 1 onion, minced
- 1 tsp. parsley, chopped
- 1 egg, beaten
- Salt and pepper to taste
- 1 tablespoon olive oil
- 4 basic chaffles
- 2 lettuce leaves
- 2 cheese slices
- 1 tablespoon dill pickles
- Ketchup
- Mayonnaise

Directions:

1. In a large bowl, combine the ground beef, onion, parsley, egg, salt and pepper.
2. Mix well.
3. Form 2 thick patties.

4. Add olive oil to the pan.
5. Place the pan over medium heat.
6. Cook the patty for 3 to 5 minutes per side or until fully cooked.
7. Place the patty on top of each chaffle.
8. Top with lettuce, cheese and pickles.
9. Squirt ketchup and mayo over the patty and veggies.
10. Top with another chaffle.

Double Choco Chaffle

Preparation Time:

5 minutes

Cooking Time:

10 minutes

Servings: 2

Ingredients:

- 1 egg
- 2 teaspoons coconut flour
- 2 tablespoons sweetener
- 1 tablespoon cocoa powder
- ¼ teaspoon baking powder
- 1 oz. cream cheese
- ½ teaspoon vanilla
- 1 tablespoon sugar-free chocolate chips

Directions:

1. Put all the ingredients in a large bowl.
2. Mix well.
3. Pour half of the mixture into the waffle maker.
4. Seal the device.
5. Cook for 4 minutes.
6. Uncover and transfer to a plate to cool.

7. Repeat the procedure to make the second chaffle.

Ketogenic Wafers with Almond Flour

Preparation time:

10 minutes

Cooking time:

10 minutes

Servings: 3

Ingredients

- 4 eggs
- 200g cream cheese
- 80g almond flour (e.g. Mea Vita almond flour)
- ½ tsp ground vanilla (e.g. Azafran vanilla powder)
- 1 teaspoon Baking powder

Directions:

1. Mix the eggs and cream cheese in a bowl, and then add the remaining ingredients.
2. Heat a chaffleiron, brush the plates with a little butter and bake 6 chaffles.

Ketogenic Wafers with Coconut Flour

Preparation time:

30 minutes

Cooking time:

10 minutes

Servings: 8

Ingredients:

- 5 eggs
- 40g coconut flour (e.g. Naturacereal organic coconut flour)
- 1 teaspoon Baking powder
- 3 tbsp unsweetened almond milk (e.g. Alpro unsweetened almond milk)
- 120g butter (e.g. from grass-fed cows)
- 1 tbsp coconut oil (e.g. Mituso organic coconut oil)

Directions:

1. The butter melts and let cool.
2. Separate the eggs and beat the egg whites until stiff.
3. In another bowl, mix egg yolk with coconut flour and baking powder and then slowly stir in the liquid butter.
4. Next add almond milk and vanilla flavor.
5. Finally carefully fold in the egg whites.

6. Heat up a chaffle iron with a little coconut oil grease. Then put the dough for 8 chaffles on the iron and bake.

Ketogenic Wafers without Flour

Preparation time:

30 minutes

Cooking time:

10 minutes

Servings: 2

Ingredients:

- 2 eggs
- 30g butter
- 50g curd cheese
- ½ tsp psyllium husk (e.g. Vita Natura Indian psyllium husk)
- 3 tbsp protein powder (e.g. ESN whey protein flavor vanilla)
- 1 tbsp coconut oil (e.g. Mituso organic coconut oil)

Directions:

1. The butter melt and let cool.
2. Then stir all the ingredients together thoroughly.
3. A chaffle maker to make hot and the coconut oil grease.
4. Add the dough in portions and even bake.

5. Depending on which protein powder you use, you can make sweet or savory chaffles.

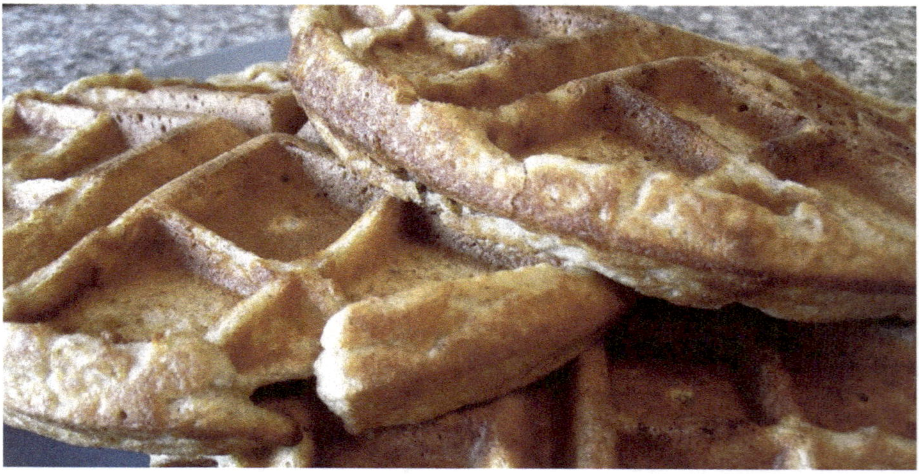

Cheese and Bacon Chaffles

Preparation time:

10 minutes

Cooking time:

5 minutes

Servings: 1

Ingredients:

- 2 egg
- 30g bacon
- 50g minced meat
- 50g grated cheese (e.g. Emmentaler)
- 1 tsp butter (e.g. from grass-fed cows)

Directions:

1. Cut the bacon into small cubes or strips and fry in a pan until crispy for 1-2 minutes.
2. Mix the egg and cheese thoroughly in a bowl.
3. Finally add the bacon and minced meat to the egg and stir.
4. Heat a chaffle iron and grease it with a little butter so that nothing sticks.

5. Pour the dough onto the chaffle iron and fry until it is as crispy as desired.

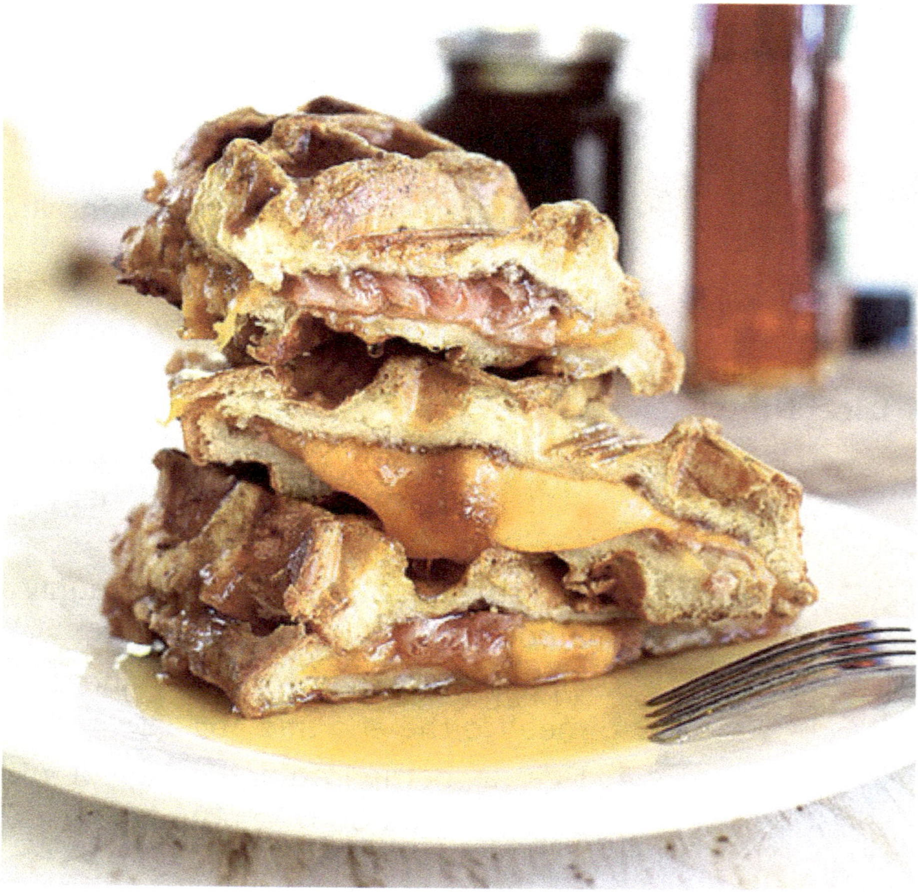

Raspberry Chaffle

Preparation time:

15 minutes

Cooking time:

5 minutes

Servings: 2

Ingredients:

- 60g raspberries (fresh or frozen)
- 1 pinch of cinnamon (e.g. Azafran Bio-Ceylon cinnamon)

Directions:

1. Simmer the raspberries in a small saucepan until you get a sauce.
2. Then add the cinnamon and pour the raspberry sauce directly and hot over the chaffles.

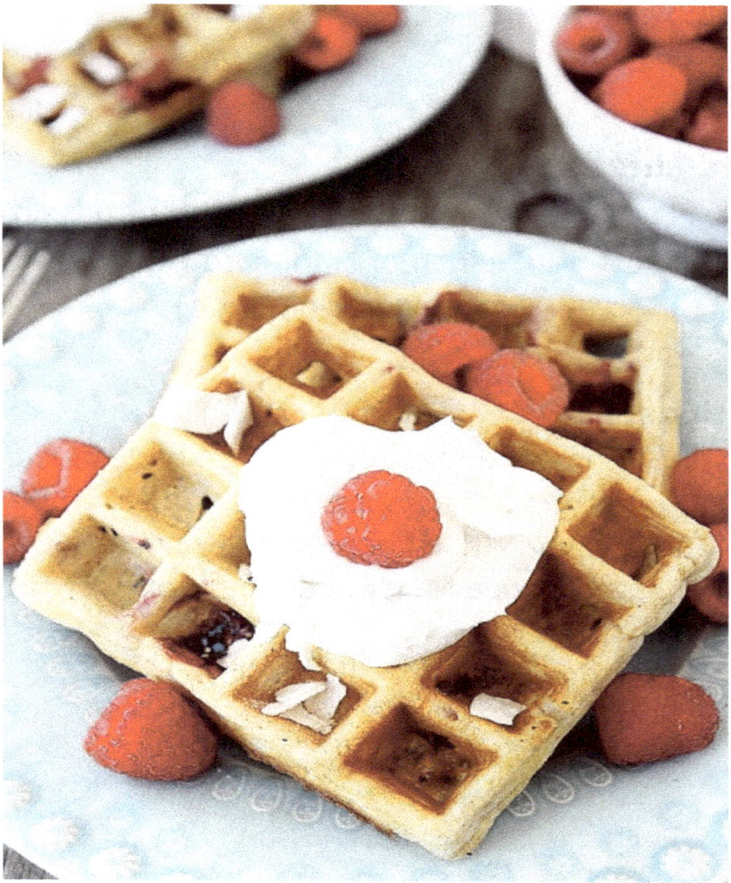

Ketogenic Chaffles

Preparation time:

25 minutes

Cooking time:

10 minutes

Servings: 6

Ingredients:

- 75 g almond flour
- 25 g vanilla protein powder
- 2 eggs
- 120 ml almond milk
- 2 tbsp coconut oil
- 1 vanilla bean
- 2 tbsp erythritol
- 1/2 tbsp baking powder

Directions:

1. Mix all the dry ingredients together.
2. Take a knife and cut the vanilla bean, scrape out the pulp with the tip of a knife and add it to the ingredients.
3. Add the eggs just like the melted coconut oil and little by little, stirring the milk.

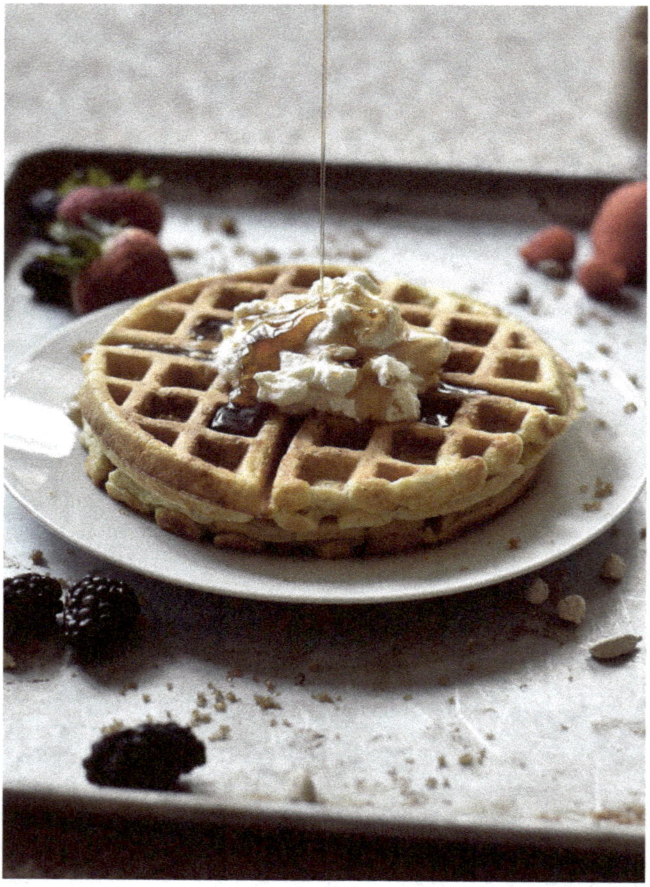

Low Carb Keto Chaffle Recipe Jalapeno Cheddar

Preparation time:

10 minutes

Cooking time:

5 minutes

Servings: 2

Ingredients:

- 80 g cream cheese
- 3 eggs
- 1 EL coconut flour
- 1 tsp psyllium seed husks
- 1 tsp baking powder
- 30 g cheddar cheese
- 1 jalapeno
- Salt
- pepper

Directions:

1. Put all the ingredients in a bowl.
2. Mix them with a hand blender until the mixture has become an evenly fine chaffle batter.
3. Turn on the chaffle maker.
4. As soon as the chaffle iron is hot enough, pour in the chaffle batter.

5. Take out the low carb chaffle if it has the right consistency for your taste.
6. Now you can serve the chaffle.

Chaffles with Raspberry Curd

Preparation time:

30 minutes

Cooking time:

10 minutes

Servings: 2

Ingredients:

- For the chaffles:
- 3 eggs (M)
- 75 g cream
- 3 tbsp psyllium husk powder
- salt
- For the curd:
- 50 g raspberries
- 200 g curd cheese (40% fat in dry matter)
- 50 g Greek yogurt
- Moreover:
- Chaffle iron
- Soft butter for greasing

Directions:

1. Mix the eggs, cream, psyllium husk powder, 1 pinch of salt and 150 ml of cold water with the whisk to smooth dough.

2. Let the dough soak for about 5 minutes.
3. In the meantime, select the raspberries, wash carefully and pat dry. Crush something in a bowl with a fork.
4. Add the curd and yogurt and mix everything until creamy.
5. Heat the chaffle iron to a medium setting. Then grease the baking surfaces thinly with the butter using a baking brush.
6. Put a quarter of the dough in the chaffle iron and bake in 3-4 minutes light brown and crispy.
7. Remove and keep warm covered on a plate.
8. Bake three more chaffles from the rest of the dough in the same way.

9. Arrange on two plates and serve with the curd.

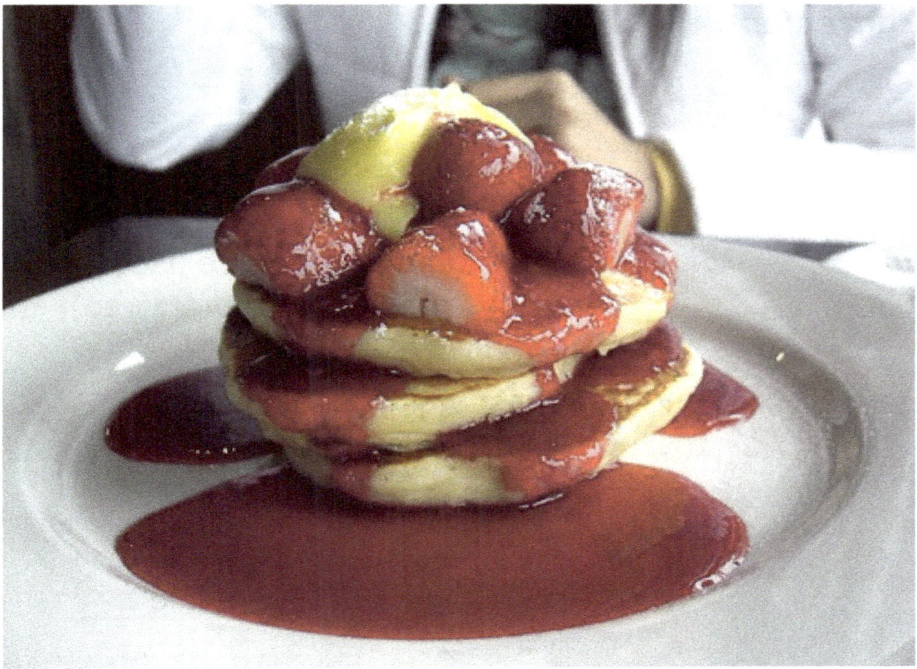

Sweet Chaffle

Preparation time:

1 minute

Cooking time:

3 minutes

Servings: 1

Ingredients:

- 2 oz cream cheese
- 1 egg
- 1 tablespoon coconut powder
- 2 tsp cocoa
- cups of sweetener (can be used between 2-3, but 2.5 is preferred)
- 1 teaspoon of vanilla
- 1/2 teaspoon baking soda
- 1 tsp cinnamon (optional)
- Coconut oil spray
- Waffle maker
- 1 teaspoon of butter (optional)

Directions:

1. Place cream cheese for 20 seconds in a microwave safe bowl and microwave. (If your cream cheese is at room temperature, this move is not required.)

2. Combine the rest of your sweet ingredients with the cream cheese in the tub.
3. Plug in your coconut oil waffle maker and spray.
4. Only spoon enough of the combined ingredients of the delicious chaffle on to the waffle maker.
5. Open your waffle maker and wait patiently, yes-it's going to be difficult.
6. Depending on your waffle maker, the exact cooking time varies.
7. We notice that in about 2 minutes most waffle makers cook the delicious chaffles.
8. Take your sweet, cooked chaffle and put it on a plate.Top with a butter slice.
9. Enjoy!

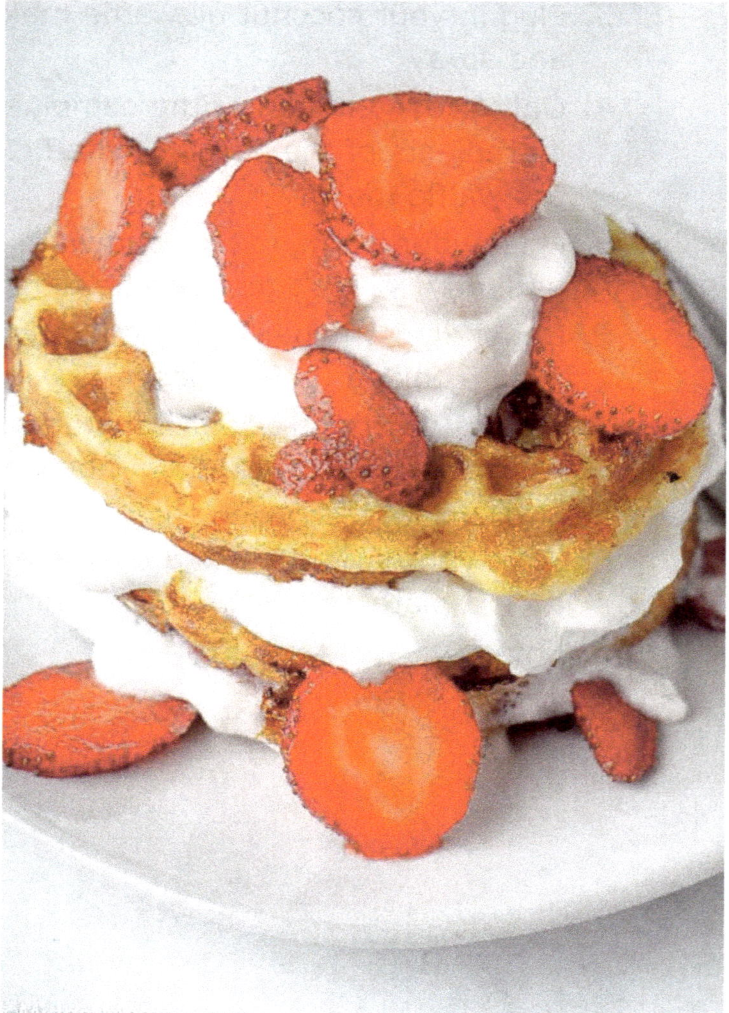

Keto Tuna Melt Chaffle

Preparation time:

5 minutes

Cooking time:

5 minutes

Servings: 2

Ingredients:

- 1/2 cup mozzarella cheese
- 1 egg
- 1 packed of tuna
- Pinch salt

Directions:

1. In a small bowl, preheat the mini waffle maker, add the egg and whip it.
2. Stir in the fish, butter, salt and combine well.
3. Add a teaspoon of cheese to the mini waffle maker for about 30 seconds before adding the mixture of the formula. When the tuna chaffle is cooked, this will allow the cheese to get crispy. This is the form I use!
4. Attach 1/2 of the waffle maker mixture and cook for at least 4 minutes.

5. Cut it and cook another 4 minutes of the last tuna chaffle.

Notes: This recipe produces two chaffles of tuna. If you use a full-size waffle maker, double the recipe.

Broccoli & Cheddar Keto Waffles

Preparation time:

5 minutes

Cooking time:

5 minutes

Servings: 1

Ingredients:

- ⅓ Raw broccoli, finely chopped 20 g
- ¼ cup cheddar cheese, shredded 28g
- 1 egg
- 1/2 teaspoon garlic powder
- 1/2 tsp dried onion
- Salt and pepper flavor
- Cooking spray

Directions:

1. To reach the temperature, insert a waffle iron.
2. Beat the egg with a fork in a small bowl.
3. Fold in broccoli, cheese, powdered garlic, onions, salt, pepper.
4. Use cooking spray as soon as the waffle iron is ready (if needed) and add the egg mixture. Cover well waffle iron and apply heat till the

light indicates that one cycle is complete.

5. Close the lid again and cook for another period.
6. When finished, gently remove the waffle iron with a tongue or fork.
7. Enjoy! Enjoy! Serve with honey, sour cream, pasture and other sauces.
8. Note: This recipe makes one or two mini waffles at full size.
9. Sprinkle with crushed cheddar cheese before and after spreading the egg mixture.

Maple Cream Cheese Icing

Preparation time:

5 minutes

Cooking time:

10 minutes

Servings: 5

Ingredients:

- 4 oz cream cheese
- 1/2 cup heavy cream
- 1/4 cup lacanto maple flavor syrup
- 1 teaspoon of vanilla essence
- 1/4 teaspoon of cinnamon

Directions:

1. Combine softened cream cheese and all other ingredients in a blender
2. Start with a pulse to combine before blending until smooth

Cinnamon Roll Chaffles With Cream Cheese Frosting

Preparation time:

5 minutes

Cooking time:

5 minutes

Servings: 1

Ingredients:

- 1 tbsp cream cheese, tender (or an alternative to sour cream or ricotta cheese)
- One large egg
- 1 teaspoon of melted butter
- 2 tablespoons almond flour (or 1 tablespoon coconut powder)
- 1/4 teaspoon baking powder
- 1 teaspoon ground cinnamon
- 1/2 teaspoon vanilla extract
- 1/4 teaspoon of cinnamon extract (or add 1/2 teaspoon of cinnamon)
- 6-8 drops of LaKanto Monkfruit extract to taste (or 2 teaspoons of granular erythritol)
- Cream cheese frosting ingredients:
- 1 oz cream cheese, softened
- 2 teaspoons powdered erythritol or taste

- 1 teaspoon of vanilla essence
- 1-2 tablespoons of heavy cream

Directions:

1. Preheat a waffle maker with a mini 4. (If you use a regular size waffle maker, double or triple the recipe.)
2. Mix all the ingredients until a smooth batter forms. (If necessary, microwave the cold cream cheese for about 5-8 seconds to soften before adding the remaining ingredients.)
3. Divide the batter into two and cook each cake for 4 minutes until well browned and crispy.
4. Two mini 4 "chaffles are made from this recipe.
5. Whisk together the whole frosting components in a small bowl and add enough heavy cream to achieve the desired consistency of spreading.
6. Spread the frosting on the warm chaffles and add extra cinnamon to sprinkle.
7. Enjoy! Enjoy!

Keto Pumpkin Cheesecake Chaffle

Preparation time:

2 minutes

Cooking time:

4 minutes

Servings: 2

Ingredients:

- Pumpkin chaffle
- 1 egg
- 1/2 cup mozzarella cheese
- 1 1/2 tbsp pumpkin puree (100% pumpkin)
- 1 tablespoon almond flour
- 1 tbsp. Of La Canto Golden Sweetener or Sweetener Choice
- 2 tsp heavy cream
- 1 teaspoon cream cheese
- 1/2 tsp pumpkin spice
- 1/2 teaspoon baking powder
- 1/2 teaspoon vanilla
- 1 teaspoon chocolate zero maple syrup or 1/8 teaspoon maple extract
- Filling
- 2 tablespoons cream cheese
- 1 tablespoon Lakant powder sweetener
- 1/4 teaspoon of vanilla essence

Directions:

1. Preheating mini waffle maker
2. In a small bowl, mix all chaffle ingredients.
3. Pour half of the chaffle mixture into the center of the waffle iron.
4. Cook for 3-5 minutes.
5. Carefully remove and repeat the second chaffle.
6. While making the filling, set it to the crunchy side.
7. With a whisk or fork, mix all the matte ingredients together.
8. Add a frost between the two chaffles. pleasant!

9. Optional: add whipped cream top, crushed pecans, chocolate zero maple syrup and more.

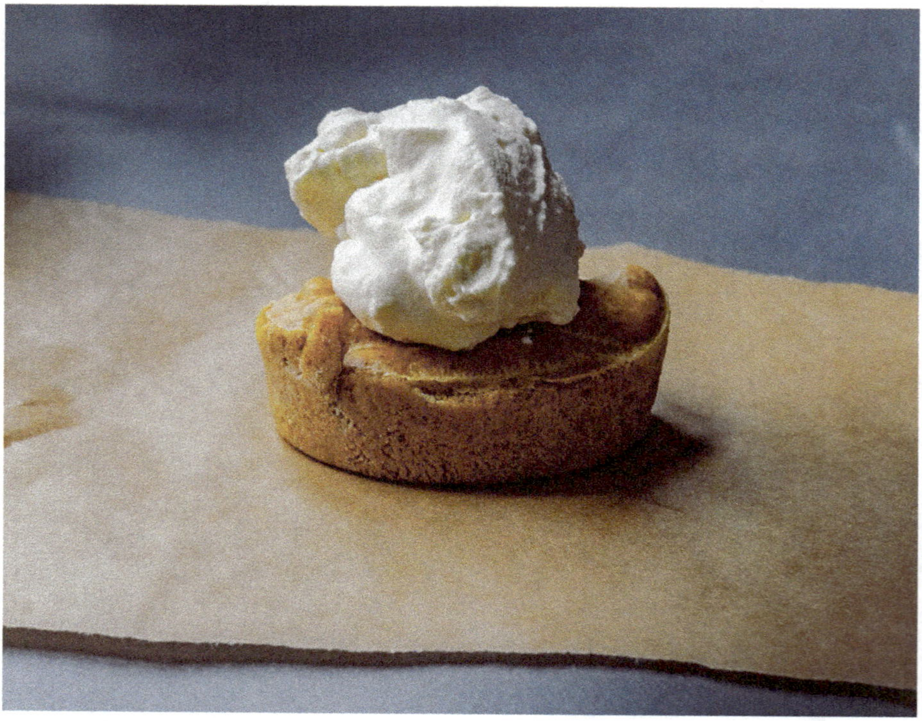

Cinnamon Apple Chaffle

Preparation time:

10 minutes

Cooking time:

5 minutes

Servings: 4

Ingredients:

- Vanilla beans sauce:
- 1/2 teaspoon monk fruit sweetener
- 1/2 teaspoon vanilla essence
- 1 egg yolk
- 1 cup whipped cream
- 1 tablespoon ghee or butter
- 2 oz cream cheese softened
- Whole vanilla bean
- Chaffle:
- 2 tablespoons coconut powder
- 1 teaspoon baking powder
- 2 tsp cinnamon
- 1/2 teaspoon monk fruit sweetener
- 3 large eggs
- ¼ cup granny smith apple skin + dice (or 1 tablespoon of natural erythritol apple flavor)
- ¾chop mozzarella cheese shredded
- ¼chop mild cheddar cheese shredded

Directions:

1. Vanilla Bean Sauce: Add heavy cream, ghee, and vanilla bean to a mild sauce.
2. Heat over medium high heat, then add sweetener and lower heat and cook for 10 minutes. Remove the vanilla bean into whipping cream and scrape the remaining vanilla seeds, then discard the bean.
3. Remove from heat and stir vigorously in egg yolk.
4. Apply cream cheese until the cheese is melted.
5. Put the vanilla sauce in a heat-safe container and cool in the refrigerator.
6. Apple Chaffle: Preheat waffle maker with low carb non-stick spray and spray generously.
7. Add egg and beat in a large mixing bowl until frothy.
8. Add vanilla and cheese and beat until thoroughly combined.
9. Whisk flour, baking powder, sweetener, and cinnamon in a small mixing bowl.
10. To egg mixture, add dry ingredients and mix until combined.
11. Fold gently in the diced apples.

12. Fluid the cooking spray from the waffle maker

13. Pour batter on low, high heat into the waffle maker and cook until the outside starts to brown–about 4 minutes.

14. Slightly cool "hole" and then top with vanilla sauce.

Peanut Butter & Jelly Sammich Chaffle

Preparation time:

5 minutes

Cooking time:

5 minutes

Servings: 2

Ingredients:

- Ingredients for chaffle
- 2 eggs
- 1/4 cup mozzarella cheese
- 1 tsp cinnamon
- 1 T confectionery
- Coconut flower 2 tsp
- 1/8 teaspoon baking powder
- 1 teaspoon of vanilla essence
- Blueberry compote ingredients
- 1 cup of washed blueberries
- 1/2 lemon peel
- Freshly squeezed 1 T lemon juice
- 1 T confectionery
- 1/8 teaspoon xanthan gum
- 2 T water

Directions:

1. Add everything except xanthan gum to a small pot.
2. Bring to a boil, lower the heat and cook for 5-10 minutes until it starts to thicken.
3. Sprinkle xanthan gum and stir well.
4. Remove from heat and cool.
5. Keep in refrigerator until ready to use.

Pandan Asian Chaffles

Preparation Time:

3 minutes

Cooking Time:

8 minutes

Servings: 2

Ingredients:

- ½ cup cheddar cheese, finely shredded
- 1 egg
- 3 drops of pandan extract
- 1 tbsp almond flour
- 1/3 tsp garlic powder

Directions:

1. Warm up your mini waffle maker.
2. Mix the egg, almond flour, garlic powder with cheese in a small bowl.
3. Add pandan extract to the cheese mixture and mix well.
4. For a crispy crust, add a teaspoon of shredded cheese to the waffle maker and cook for 30 seconds.
5. Then, pour the mixture into the waffle maker and cook for 5 minutes or until crispy.
6. Repeat with remaining batter.

7. Serve with fried chicken wings with bbq sauce and enjoy!

Ham and Jalapenos Chaffle

Preparation Time:

5 minutes

Cooking Time:

9 minutes

Servings: 3

Ingredients:

- 2 lbs cheddar cheese, finely grated
- 2 large eggs
- ½ jalapeno pepper, finely grated
- 2 ounces ham steak
- 1 medium scallion
- 2 tsp coconut flour

Directions:

1. Shred the cheddar cheese using a fine grater.
2. Deseed the jalapeno and grate using the same grater.
3. Finely chop the scallion and ham.
4. Pour all the ingredients in a medium bowl and mix well.
5. Spray your waffle iron with cooking spray and heat for 3 minutes.
6. Pour 1/4 of the batter mixture into the waffle iron.
7. Cook for 3 minutes, until crispy around the edges.

8. Remove the waffles from the heat and repeat until all the batter is finished.
9. Once done, allow them to cool to room temperature and enjoy.

Hot Ham Chaffles

Preparation Time:

5 minutes

Cooking Time:

4 minutes

Servings: 2

Ingredients:

- ½ cup mozzarella cheese, shredded
- 1 egg
- ¼ cup ham, chopped
- ¼ tsp salt
- 2 tbsp mayonnaise
- 1 tsp Dijon mustard

Directions:

1. Preheat your waffle iron.
2. In the meantime, add the egg in a small mixing bowl and whisk.
3. Add in the ham, cheese, and salt. Mix to combine.
4. Scoop half the mixture using a spoon and pour into the hot waffle iron.
5. Close and cook for 4 minutes.
6. Remove the waffle and place on a large plate. Repeat the process with the remaining batter.

7. In a separate small bowl, add the mayo and mustard. Mix together until smooth.
8. Slice the waffles in quarters and use the mayo mixture as the dip.

Cheese-free Breakfast Chaffle

Preparation Time:

4 minutes

Cooking Time:

12 minutes

Servings: 1

Ingredients:

- 1 egg
- ½ cup almond milk ricotta, finely shredded.
- 1 tbsp almond flour
- 2 tbsp butter

Directions:

1. Mix the egg, almond flour and ricotta in a small bowl.
2. Separate the chaffle batter into two and cook each for 4 minutes.
3. Melt the butter and pour on top of the chaffles.
4. Put them back in the pan and cook on each side for 2 minutes.
5. Remove from the pan and allow them sit for 2 minutes.
6. Enjoy while still crispy.

Bacon Chaffle Omelettes

Preparation Time:

5 minutes

Cooking Time:

10 minutes

Servings: 2

Ingredients:

- 2 slices bacon, raw
- 1 egg
- 1 tsp maple extract, optional
- 1 tsp all spices

Directions:

1. Put the bacon slices in a blender and turn it on.
2. Once ground up, add in the egg and all spices. Go on blending until liquefied.
3. Heat your waffle maker on the highest setting and spray with non-stick cooking spray.
4. Pour half the omelette into the waffle maker and cook for 5 minutes max.
5. Remove the crispy omelette and repeat the same steps with rest batter.
6. Enjoy warm.

Avocado Chaffle Toast

Preparation Time:

4 minutes

Cooking Time:

8 minutes

Servings: 2

Ingredients:

- ½ avocado
- 1 egg
- ½ cup cheddar cheese, finely shredded
- 1 tbsp almond flour
- 1 tsp lemon juice, fresh
- Salt, ground pepper to taste
- Parmesan cheese, finely shredded for garnishing

Directions:

1. Warm up your mini waffle maker.
2. Mix the egg, almond flour with cheese in a small bowl.
3. For a crispy crust, add a teaspoon of shredded cheese to the waffle maker and cook for 30 seconds.
4. Then, pour the mixture into the waffle maker and cook for 5 minutes or until crispy.

5. Repeat with remaining batter.
6. Mash avocado with a fork until well combined and add lemon juice, salt, pepper
7. Top each chaffle with avocado mixture. Sprinkle with parmesan and enjoy!

Crab Chaffles

Preparation Time:

10 minutes

Cooking Time:

25 minutes

Servings: 6

Ingredients:

- 1 lb crab meat
- 1/3 cup Panko breadcrumbs
- 1 egg
- 2 tbsp fat greek yogurt
- 1 tsp Dijon mustard
- 2 tbsp parsley and chives, fresh
- 1 tsp Italian seasoning
- 1 lemon, juiced
- Salt, pepper to taste

Directions:

1. Preheat the waffle maker
2. Mix all the ingredients in a small mixing bowl, except crab meat.
3. Add the meat. Mix well.
4. Form the mixture into round patties.
5. Cook 1 patty for 3 minutes.
6. Remove it and repeat the process with the remaining crab chaffle mixture.

7. Once ready, remove and enjoy warm.

Jalapeno Pepper Chaffle

Preparation time:

10 minutes

Cooking time:

20 minutes

Servings: 4

Ingredients:

- 4 slices of bacon, cooked, crumbled
- 3 tablespoon coconut flour
- 1 jalapeno pepper, deseeded, sliced
- 1 jalapeno pepper, deseeded, diced
- 1 teaspoon baking powder
- ¼ teaspoon of sea salt
- 1 cup / 115 grams shredded cheddar cheese
- 3 eggs, at room temperature
- 1 cup / 225 grams cream cheese, softened

Directions:

1. Take a non-stick waffle iron, plug it in, select the medium or medium-high heat setting and let it preheat until ready to use; it could also be

indicated with an indicator light changing its color.

2. Meanwhile, prepare the batter and for this, take a large bowl, add flour in it, stir in baking powder, and salt until mixed.
3. Take another bowl, place cream cheese in it, and beat with an electric mixer until fluffy.
4. Crack eggs in a separate bowl, beat with an electric mixer until fluffy, then add cheddar cheese and ½ cup of beaten cream cheese and continue beating until combined.
5. Add flour mixture into egg-cream cheese mixture, beat with an electric mixer until incorporated, and then fold in diced peppers.
6. Use a ladle to pour one-fourth of the prepared batter into the heated waffle iron in a spiral direction, starting from the edges, then shut the lid and cook for 5 minutes or more until solid and nicely browned; the cooked waffle will look like a cake.
7. When done, transfer chaffles to a plate with a silicone spatula and repeat with the remaining batter.

8. Let chaffles stand for some time until crispy, then top with bacon, jalapeno slices and remaining cream cheese and then serve.

Avocado Toast Chaffle

Preparation time:

12 minutes

Cooking time:

6 minutes

Servings: 2

Ingredients:

- Egg: 2
- Whole avocado: 1 whole
- Salt: ¼ teaspoon or as per your taste
- Cheddar cheese: 1 cup
- Lemon juice: 1 teaspoon
- Black pepper: ¼ teaspoon or as per your taste

Directions:

1. Prepare a mix of peeled and cut avocados into a bowl, add some salt, pepper and lemon juice then mash with a fork.
2. Quickly, preheat a mini-sized waffle and grease it. In another mixing bowl, prepare a mix of cheddar cheese with beaten eggs.
3. Combine the mixture and pour into the lower side of the waffle maker.
4. With the lid closed, cook for 5 minutes to a crunch. Once timed out, take out waffles and allow sitting for a minute.

5. Apply mashed avocado on the chaffles and serve in a plate.

Mc Griddle Chaffle

Preparation time:

12 minutes

Cooking time:

6 minutes

Servings: 2

Ingredients:

- Egg: 2
- Maple Syrup: 2 tablespoon (sugar-free)
- American cheese: 2 slices
- Swerve/Monk fruit: 2 tablespoon
- Mozzarella Cheese: 1½ cup (shredded)
- Sausage patty: 2

Directions:

1. Quickly preheat a mini-sized waffle maker and grease with oil.
2. Using a mixing bowl, prepare a mix containing shredded mozzarella cheese, beaten eggs,
3. Monk fruit/Swerve and maple syrup and mix into a homogenous state.
4. With a closed lid, heat the waffle for 5 minutes to a crunch.
5. Once timed out, remove the chaffle from the waffle maker.
6. Repeat for the remaining chaffles mixture.

7. Following the instructions on the pack, prepare the sausage patty with a garnish of sliced cheese when removing from heat.
8. Arrange two chaffles with sliced cheese in between and serve hot.

Cinnamon Swirl Chaffle

Preparation time:

12 minutes

Cooking time:

6 minutes

Servings: 2

Ingredients:

- Icing
- Butter: 2 tablespoons unsalted butter
- Cream cheese: 2 oz softened
- Vanilla: 1 teaspoon
- Splenda: 2 tablespoons
- Chaffle
- Egg: 2
- Almond flour: 2 tablespoons
- Cinnamon: 2 teaspoons
- Splenda: 2 tablespoons
- Cream Cheese: 2 oz softened
- Vanilla Extract: 2 teaspoons
- Vanilla extract: 2 teaspoons
- Cinnamon Drizzle
- Splenda: 2 tablespoons
- Cinnamon: 2 teaspoons
- Butter: 1 tablespoon

Directions:

1. Preheat and grease a waffle maker.
2. Prepare a combined mixture of all ingredients, evenly mixed and pour into the waffle maker.
3. Cook for 4 minutes till chaffles turns crispy, and then set aside.
4. Using a mixing bowl, prepare a mix of all ingredients for icing and the cinnamon drizzle, then heat using a microwave for 12 seconds to soften.
5. Pour heated icing and cinnamon on the cool chaffles to enjoy.

Cinnamon Chaffle

Preparation time:

18 minutes

Cooking time:

12 minutes

Servings: 2

Ingredients:

- Egg: 1
- Vanilla extract: 1 tablespoon
- Baking powder: ½ teaspoon
- Mozzarella: ½ cup
- Almond flour: 1 tablespoon

Directions:

1. Quickly preheat a mini-sized waffle maker and grease with oil.
2. Using a mixing bowl, prepare a mix containing all the ingredients.
3. With a closed lid, heat the waffle for 5 minutes to a crunch.
4. Once timed out, remove the chaffle from the waffle maker.
5. Repeat for the remaining chaffles mixture.
6. Serve hot with any of your favorite toppings.

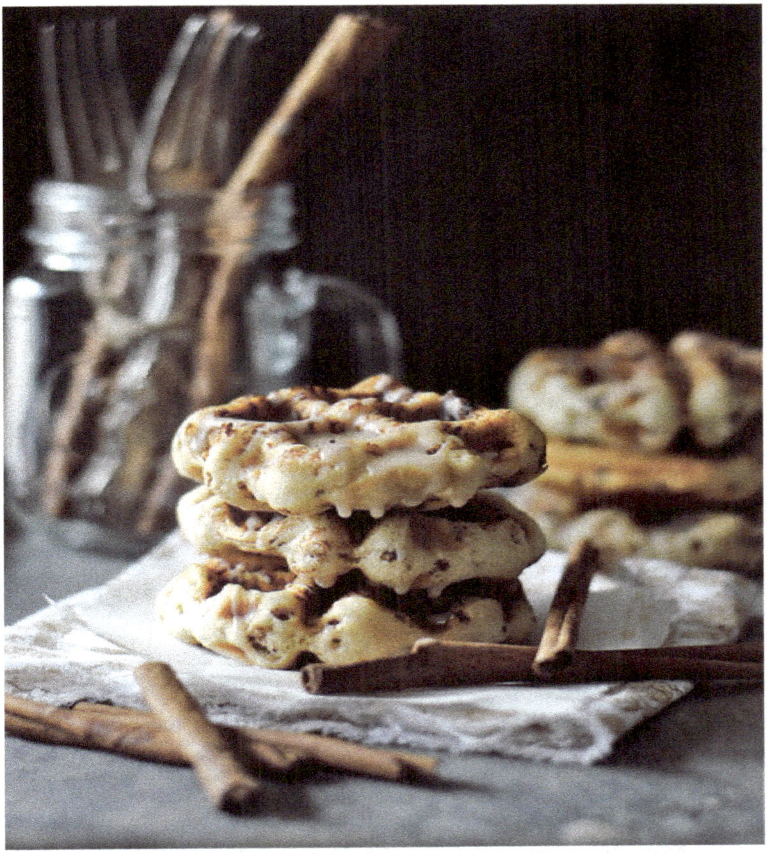

Japanese Styled Breakfast Chaffle

Preparation time:

12 minutes

Cooking time:

6 minutes

Servings: 2

Ingredients:

- Egg: 1
- Bacon: 1 slice
- Green onion: 1 stalk
- Mozzarella Cheese: 1/2 cup (shredded)
- Kewpie Mayo: 2 tablespoon

Directions:

1. Preheat and grease the waffle maker.
2. Using a mixing bowl prepare a mix containing kewpie mayo with beaten egg, then add in ½ chopped green onion with the other ½ kept aside, and ¼ inches of cut bacon into the mixture.
3. Mix evenly. Sprinkle the base of the waffle maker with 1/8 cup of shredded mozzarella and pour in the mixture, then top with more shredded mozzarella.
4. With a closed lid, heat the waffle for 5 minutes to a crunch and then remove the chaffle and allow cooking for a few minutes.

5. Repeat for the remaining chaffles mixture to make more batter.
6. Serve by garnishing the chaffle with the leftover chopped green onions.
7. Enjoy.

Keto Strawberry Chaffle

Preparation time:

Cooking time:

Servings:

Ingredients:

- 1 egg
- 1/4 cup mozzarella cheese
- 1 tablespoonful cream cheese
- 1/4 teaspoonful baking powder
- 2 sliced strawberries
- 1 teaspoonfull strawberry extract

Directions:

1. Preheat waffle maker.
2. In a little bowl, beat the egg.
3. Add the rest of the ingredients.
4. The waffle maker is sprayed with non stick cooking spray.
5. Divide the mix into two equal parts.
6. Cook a portion of the mix for around 4 minutes or until golden brown colored.
7. Homemade made whipped cream: 1 cup whipping cream, 1 teaspoonful vanilla, 1 tablespoonful monkfruit confectioners mix.
8. Whip until it forms a mix.

Keto Crunchy Chaffle

Preparation time:

15 minutes

Cooking time:

8 minutes

Ingredients:

- 2 Large Eggs
- 1/2 Cup Shredded Mozarella Cheese (pressed firmly)
- 1/2 teaspoon Baking Powder
- 1 Tablespoon Erythritol (powder), or sweetener (however powder is most ideal)
- 1/2 teaspoon Vanilla Extract

Directions:

1. Heat You Waffle Iron on the high heat setting.
2. I used a 7 inch waffle Iron and this formula fits nicely for one huge waffle.
3. If you have a smaller waffle iron, you will need to divide the recipe into two waffles.
4. Put all ingredients into a Bullet or a Blender and blend for 10 seconds.

5. Pour the mix into a very hot and dry waffle Iron. It will look thin once poured but have no fear it significantly increases in size when it cooks (and you'll need to keep an eye on it to avoid overflow when cooking!).
6. Let the waffle to Cook for 3-4 minutes or much more! The waffle is done once the entire waffle is golden dark-colored, which takes longer than a normal waffle would.
7. You can use a fork to flip your waffle to ensure that each side has even colors if it doesn't look done after some time.
8. Let waffle cool for 3-4 minutes before eating since it may become brown on cooling

9. Serve with gobs of grass-fed butter and sugar-free syrup, or whatever topping you want.

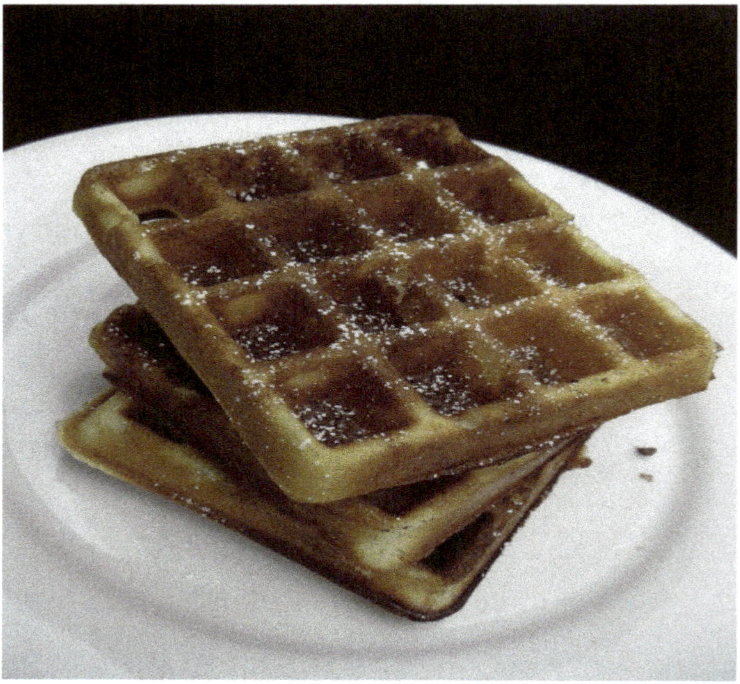

Keto Silver Dollar Pancakes

Preparation time:

10 minutes

Cooking time:

5 minutes

Ingredients:

- (3) Eggs
- 1/2 Cup (105 G) Cottage Cheese
- 1/3 Cup (37.33 G) Superfine Almond Flour
- 1/4 Cup (62.5 G) Unsweetened Almond Milk
- 2 Tablespoons Truvia
- Vanilla Extract
- 1 Teaspoon Baking Powder
- Cooking Oil Spray

Directions:

1. place ingredients in a blender in the order listed above.
2. Mix until you have a smooth, fluid batter.
3. Heat a nonstick pan on medium-high temperature. Spray with oil or margarine.
4. Place 2 tablespoons of batter at once to make little, dollar hotcakes. This is

an extremely fluid, sensitive batter so don't

5. attempt to make big pancakes with this one as they won't flip over easily.
6. Cook every pancake until the top of the hotcake has made little air pockets and the air pockets have vanished, around 1-2 minutes.
7. Using a spatula, tenderly loosen the pan cake, and afterward flip over.
8. Make the remainder of the pancakes and serve hot.

Keto Chaffle Waffle

Preparation time:

Cooking time:

Ingredients:

- 1 egg
- ½ cup of shredded mozzarella cheese
- 1 ½ table-spoon of almond flour
- Pinch of baking powder
- Equipment:
- Waffle Maker
- Shredder (to shred solid mozzarella cheese)

Directions:

1. Start by turning your waffle maker on and preheating it. During the time of pre-heating, in a bowl, whisk the egg and shredded mozzarella cheese together. If you do not have shredded mozzarella cheese, you can use the shredder to shred your cheese, Then add the almond powder and baking powder to the bowl and whisk them until the mixture is consistent.
2. Then pour the mixture onto the waffle machine.

3. Make sure you pour it to the center of the mixture will come out of the edges on closing the machine.
4. Close the machine and let the waffles cook until golden brown.
5. Then you can serve your tasty chaffle waffles.

Nutrition: Calories 320 Carbohydrates 2.9 g Protein 21.5 g Fat 24.3g

Keto Chaffle Topped With Salted Caramel Syrup

Preparation time:

15 minutes

Cooking time:

10 minutes

Ingredients:

- 1 egg
- ½ cup of mozzarella cheese
- ¼ cup of cream
- 2 tablespoon of collagen powder
- 1 ½ tablespoon of almond flour
- 1 ½ tablespoon of unsalted butter
- Pinch of salt
- ¾ tablespoon of powdered erythritol
- Pinch of baking powder

Directions:

1. Begin by preheating your waffle machine by switching it on and turning the heat to medium.
2. Whisk together the chaffle ingredients that include the egg, mozzarella cheese, almond flour, and baking powder.
3. Pour the mixture on the waffle machine. Let it cook until golden

brown. You can make up to two chaffles with this method.

4. To make the caramel syrup, you will need to turn on the flame under a pan to medium heat Melt the unsalted butter on the pan.
5. Then turn the heat low and add collagen powder and erythritol to the pan and whisk them.
6. Gradually add the cream and remove from heat.
7. Then add the salt and continue to whisk.
8. Pour the syrup onto the chaffle, and here you go.

Nutrition: 605 calories 45g fat 48g protein g of carbohydrates

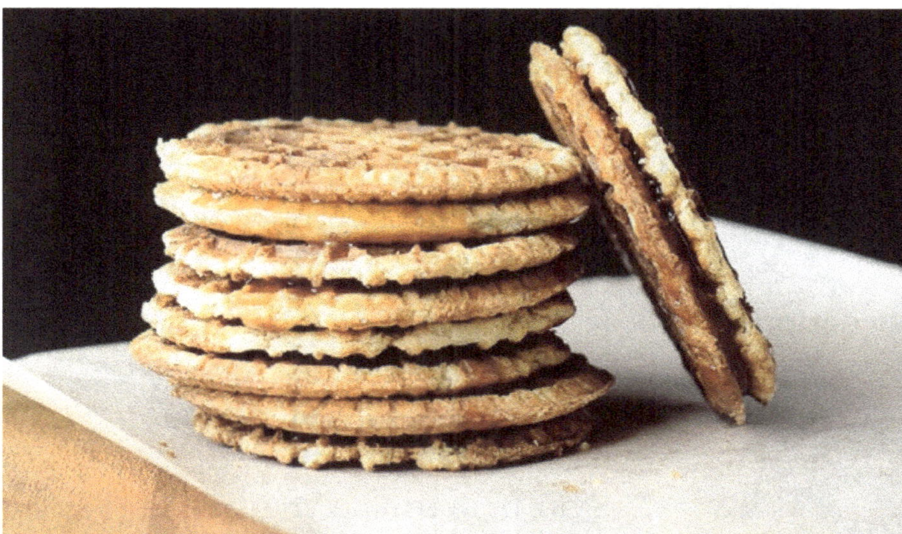

Keto Chaffle Bacon Sandwich

Preparation time:

15 minutes

Cooking time:

10 minutes

Ingredients:

- 1 egg
- ½ cup of shredded mozzarella cheese
- 2 Tablespoon of coconut flour
- 2 strips of pork or beef bacon
- 1 slice of any type of cheese
- 2 tablespoon of coconut oil

Directions:

1. To make the chaffle, you will be following the typical recipe for making a chaffle.
2. Start by warming your waffle machine to medium heat. In a bowl, beat 1 egg, ½ cup of mozzarella cheese, and almond flour.
3. Pour the mixture on the waffle machine.
4. Let it cook until it is golden brown.
5. Then remove in a plate.
6. Warm coconut oil in a pan over medium heat. Then place the bacon strips in the pan.

7. Cook until crispy over medium heat.
8. Assemble the bacon and cheese on the chaffle.

Nutrition: Calories 580 Fat 52 g Carbohydrates 3g

Crispy Zucchini Chaffle

Preparation time:

15 minutes

Cooking time:

5 minutes

Ingredients:

- 2 eggs
- 1 fresh zucchini
- 1 cup of shredded or grated cheddar cheese
- 2 pinch of salt
- 1 tablespoon of onion (chopped)
- 1 clove of garlic

Directions:

1. Start by preheating the waffle maker to medium heat.
2. The best way to make a chaffle is to make it with layering.
3. Start by dicing onions and mashing the garlic.
4. Then use the grater to grate the zucchini.
5. Then take a bowl and add 2 eggs and add the grated zucchini to the bowl.
6. Also, add the onions, salt, and garlic for extra flavor.

7. You can also add other herbs to give your zaffle a crispy more flavor. Then sprinkle ½ cup of cheese on top of the waffle machine.
8. Add the mixture from the bowl to the waffle machine. Add the remaining cheese on top of the waffle machine and close the waffle machine. Make sure the waffle cooks for about 3 to 5 minutes until it turns golden brown.
9. By the layering method, you will achieve the perfect crisp. Take out your zucchini chaffles and serve them hot and fresh.
10. Equipment:
11. Waffle maker
12. Grater to grate the cheese

Nutrition: Calories 170 Fat 12g Carbohydrates 4g Protein 11g

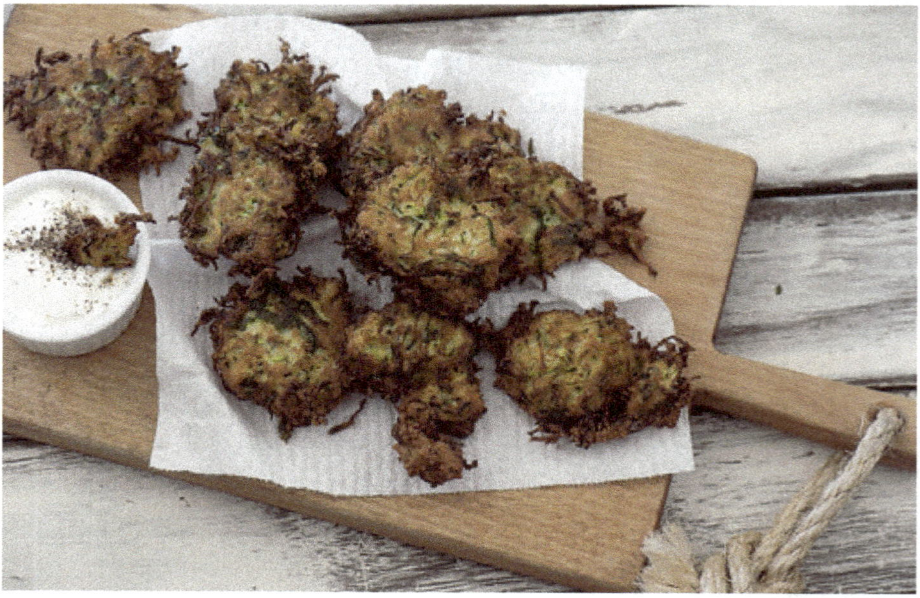

Peanut Butter Chaffle

Preparation time:

15 minutes

Cooking time:

10 minutes

Ingredients:

- 1 egg
- ½ cup of cheddar cheese
- 2 tablespoon of peanut butter
- Few drops of vanilla extract

Directions:

1. To make deliciously tasting peanut butter chaffles. Take a grater and grate some cheddar cheese.
2. Add one egg, cheddar cheese, 2 tablespoon of peanut butter, and a few drops of vanilla extract.
3. Beat these ingredients together until the batter is consistent enough.
4. Then sprinkle some shredded cheese as a base on the waffle maker.
5. Pour the mixture on top of the waffle machine.
6. Sprinkle more cheese on top of the mixture and close the waffle machine.

7. Ensure that the waffle is cooked thoroughly for about a few minutes until they are golden brown.
8. Then remove it and enjoy your deliciously cooked chaffles.

Equipment:

Waffle maker

Grater

Nutrition: 363 Calories 29 g of Fat 22 g of Protein 4 g of Carbohydrates

Morning Chaffles With Berries

Preparation Time:

5 Minutes

Cooking Time:

5 Minutes

Servings: 4

Ingredients:

- 1 Cup Egg Whites
- 1 cup cheddar cheese, shredded
- ¼ cup almond flour
- ¼ cup heavy cream

Topping:

- 4 Oz. Raspberries
- 4 Oz. Strawberries.
- 1 Oz. Keto Chocolate Flakes
- 1 Oz. Feta Cheese.

Directions:

1. Preheat your square waffle maker and grease with cooking spray.
2. Beat egg white in a small bowl with flour.
3. Add shredded cheese to the egg whites and flour mixture and mix well.
4. Add cream and cheese tothe egg mixture.
5. Pour Chaffles batter in a waffle maker and close the lid.

6. Cook chaffles for about 4 minutes until crispy and brown.
7. Carefully remove chaffles from the maker.
8. Serve with berries, cheese, and chocolate on top.
9. Enjoy!

Chaffles Breakfast Bowl

Preparation Time:

10 Minutes

Cooking Time:

5 Minutes

Servings: 2

Ingredients:

- 1 Egg
- 1/2 cup cheddar cheese shredded
- pinch of Italian seasoning
- 1 tbsp. pizza sauce

Topping:

- 1/2 Avocado Sliced
- 2 Eggs Boiled
- 1 Tomato, Halves
- 4 Oz. Fresh Spinach Leaves

Directions:

1. Preheat yourwaffle maker and grease with cooking spray.
2. Crack an egg in a small bowl and beat with Italian seasoning and pizza sauce.
3. Add shredded cheese to the egg and spices mixture.
4. Pour 1 tbsp. shredded cheese in a waffle maker and cook for 30 sec.

5. Pour Chaffles batter inthe waffle maker and close the lid.
6. Cook chaffles for about 4 minutes until crispy and brown.
7. Carefully remove chaffles from the maker.
8. Serve on the bed of spinach with boil egg, avocado slice, and tomatoes.
9. Enjoy!

Crispy Chaffles With Sausage

Preparation Time:

5 Min

Cooking Time:

10 Min

Servings: 2

Ingredients:

- 1/2 cup cheddar cheese
- 1/2 tsp. baking powder
- 1/4 cup egg whites
- 2 tsp. pumpkin spice
- 1 egg, whole
- 2 chicken sausage
- 2 slice bacon
- salt and pepper to taste
- 1 tsp. avocado oil

Directions:

1. Mix together all ingredients in a bowl.
2. Allow batter to sit while waffle iron warms.
3. Spray waffle iron with nonstick spray.
4. Pour batter in the waffle maker and cook according to the directions of the manufacturer.

5. Meanwhile, heat oil in a pan and fry the egg, according to your choice and transfer it toa plate.
6. In the same pan, fry bacon slice and sausage on medium heat for about 2-3 minutes until cooked.
7. Once chaffles are cooked thoroughly, remove them from the maker.
8. Serve with fried egg, bacon slice, sausages and enjoy!

Mini Breakfast Chaffles

Preparation Time:

5 Minutes

Cooking Time:

15 Minutes

Servings: 3

Ingredients:

- 6 tsp coconut flour
- 1 tsp stevia
- 1/4 tsp baking powder
- 2 eggs
- 3 oz. cream cheese
- 1/2. tsp vanilla extract

Topping:

- 1 egg
- 6 slice bacon
- 2 oz. Raspberries for topping
- 2 oz. Blueberries for topping
- 2 oz. Strawberries for topping

Directions:

1. Heat up your square waffle maker and grease with cooking spray.
2. Mix together coconut flour, stevia, egg, baking powder, cheese and vanilla in mixing bowl.

3. Pour ½ of chaffles mixture in a waffle maker.
4. Close the lid and cook the chaffles for about 3-5 minutes.
5. Meanwhile, fry bacon slices in pan on medium heat for about 2-3 minutes until cooked and transfer themto plate.
6. In the same pan, fry eggs one by one in the leftover grease of bacon.
7. Once chaffles are cooked, carefully transferthem toplate.
8. Serve with fried eggs and bacon slice and berries on top.
9. Enjoy!

Crispy Chaffles With Egg & Asparagus

Preparation Time:

5 Minutes

Cooking Time:

10 Minutes

Servings: 1

Ingredients:

- 1 egg
- 1/4 cup cheddar cheese
- 2 tbsps. almond flour
- ½ tsp. baking powder

Topping:

- 1 egg
- 4-5 stalks asparagus
- 1 tsp avocado oil

Directions:

1. Preheat waffle maker to medium-high heat.
2. Whisk together egg, mozzarella cheese, almond flour, and baking powder
3. Pour chaffles mixture into the center of the waffle iron. Close the waffle maker and let cook for 3-5 minutes or until waffle is golden brown and set.

4. Remove chaffles from the waffle maker and serve.
5. Meanwhile, heat oil in a nonstick pan.
6. Once the pan is hot, fry asparagus for about 4-5 minutes until golden brown.
7. Poach the egg in boil water for about 2-3 minutes.
8. Once chaffles are cooked, remove from the maker.
9. Serve chaffles with the poached egg and asparagus.

Coconut Chaffles

Preparation Time:

5 Minutes

Cooking Time:

5 Minutes

Servings: 2

Ingredients:

- 1 egg
- 1 oz. cream cheese,
- 1 oz. cheddar cheese
- 2 tbsps. coconut flour
- 1 tsp. stevia
- 1 tbsp. coconut oil, melted
- 1/2 tsp. coconut extract
- 2 eggs, soft boil for serving

Directions:

1. Heat you mini Dash waffle maker and grease with cooking spray.
2. Mix together all chaffles ingredients in a bowl.
3. Pour chaffle batter in a preheated waffle maker.
4. Close the lid.
5. Cook chaffles for about 2-3 minutes until golden brown.

6. Serve with boil egg and enjoy!

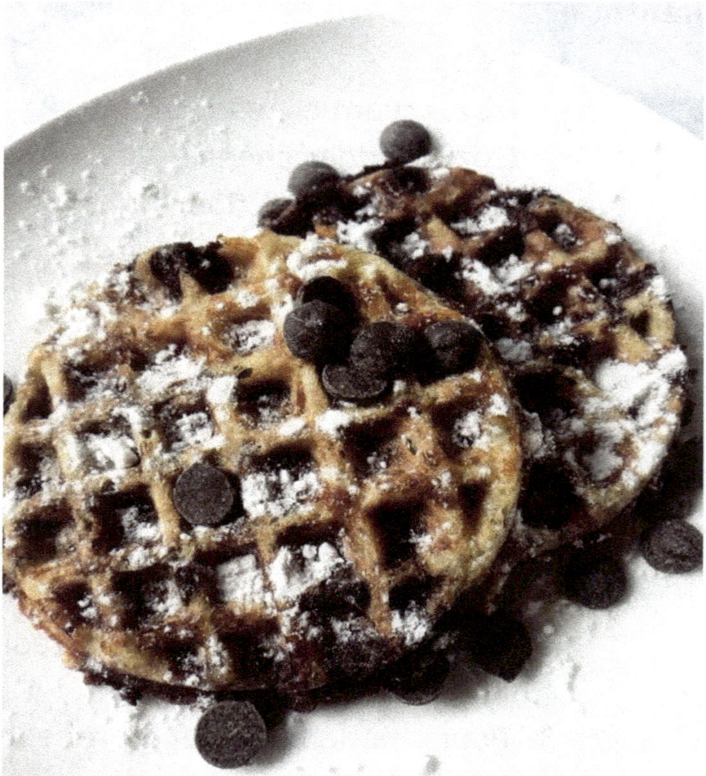

CPSIA information can be obtained
at www.ICGtesting.com
Printed in the USA
BVHW091123210621
610125BV00004B/1023

9 781803 177762